SAUNAS SIMPLIFIED

COURTNEY CARTER

AUTHOR'S NOTE

Given the overwhelming number of sources, experts, articles, and podcasts discussing saunas, you might wonder why you should listen to me. Well, here's the deal, I'm not claiming to be an expert, and I won't pretend to be one. But what I can tell you is that I've done my homework and gathered insights from real experts, scientific studies, and published articles on sauna usage.

This book aims to give you quick facts on saunas so you don't have to go through all the digging I did to find the truth. The scientific methods and jargon can be confusing and sometimes, quite frankly, boring. Our goal is to cut through the noise and get to the good stuff.

CONTENTS

Part 3: Disadvantages

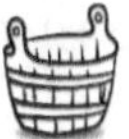

INTRODUCTION

Saunas have a rich history and are cherished in many cultures worldwide. While the exact origins of saunas are debated, their therapeutic benefits have been recognized for thousands of years. Finland, in particular, has a deep connection to saunas. In recent decades, saunas have finally gained the attention they deserve. With that, there has also been an influx of false marketing claims.

Rest assured, all the guidance, benefits, and insights shared in this book are sourced directly from reputable health experts, such as:

- Jari Laukkanen, MD, PhD - a Finnish cardiologist who has extensively researched the health benefits of sauna use.

- Rhonda Patrick, PhD - a biomedical scientist who has published research on the effects of heat stress on the body and has discussed the benefits of sauna use in her work.

This book will explore the different aspects of saunas and their potential health benefits from trusted experts, scientific studies, and evidence-based information.

PART 1
BACKGROUND

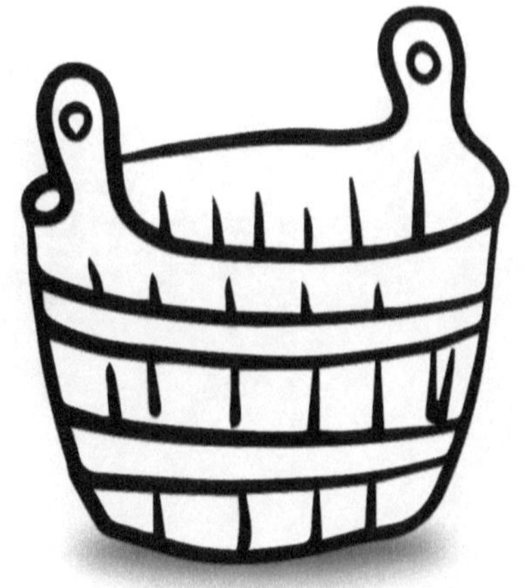

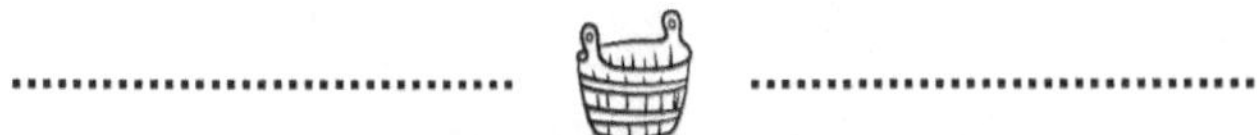

CHAPTER ONE

HISTORY

Honestly, I had a tough time finding a definitive answer for when saunas were invented and by whom. Some sources suggest they may date back 2,000 years, while others say 10,000 years. Whether it's Turkish hammams, Russian banyas, Native American sweat lodges, or Finnish saunas, heat therapy spans many different origins and cultures.

Now, when it comes to Finland, saunas hold a special place in their hearts.

- The word "sauna" is believed to have originated from the Finnish word "savu," which means "smoke." Smoke refers to the traditional method of heating saunas by burning wood.

- Sauna culture is rooted in Finnish society, with an estimated three million saunas in the country, for a population of five million. There's even a Ferris wheel with a sauna and an in-store sauna at Burger King in Helsinki.
- In the 1960s, the Finnish-American community in the upper Midwest helped to popularize sauna use in the United States. Many Finnish immigrants built saunas in their homes and passed down the tradition to subsequent generations.
- The sauna experience gained popularity in America in the 1970s as part of the broader interest in wellness and alternative therapies. The counterculture movement embraced the sauna as a natural, holistic form of health care.

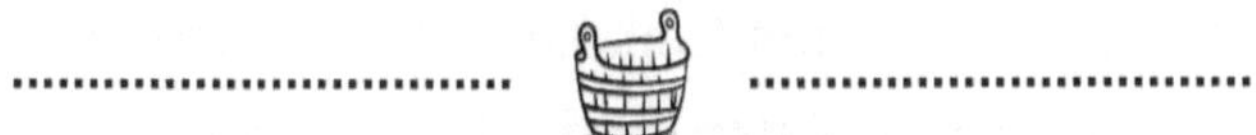

CHAPTER TWO

TEMPERATURE

Sauna temperatures play a critical role in determining the therapeutic and physiological benefits. Begin at a lower temperature and gradually increase to find what works for you. Comfort is key, so listen to your body and adjust accordingly.

- Traditional dry saunas heat the air to create a hot environment in wood-lined rooms. In a traditional Finnish sauna, the optimal range is between 176°F (80°C) and 194°F (90°C) (Kukkonen-Harjula et al., 2006). They typically use electric heaters or wood-burning stoves and generate steam, known as "löyly," by pouring water onto heated rocks. Air humidity ranges from 10-20%. Purists consider this the only "true" sauna.

- Infrared saunas are a bit different. Unlike traditional saunas that heat the air around you, infrared saunas use radiant heat, which warms your body directly. With a range of 113°F (45°C) to 140°F (60°C), they don't get as hot as traditional dry saunas (Beever, 2009).
- Steam rooms (sometimes called wet saunas) are generally kept at temperatures ranging from 100°F (38°C) to 120°F (49°C) but can feel hotter because humidity can reach 100% (Pilch et al., 2014).

CHAPTER THREE

GUIDELINES

To maximize the benefits and safety of your sauna sessions, follow these essential guidelines, including expert advice on the ideal sauna type and temperature.

- Prioritize traditional dry saunas at a minimum temperature of 174°F. (See Chapter Four for more background).
- An old Finnish guideline is the 'Rule of 200' for optimal comfort in a traditional sauna. Meaning that the temperature plus the humidity should equal 200°F. In other words, if the sauna is 170°F, the humidity levels should be 30%.
- Sauna four to seven times weekly for about 5-30

minutes each session. Most (not all...) benefits are dose-dependent, meaning the more that you sauna, the better. Longer sessions elicit more robust protective effects.

- Drink two to four glasses of water after a sauna.
- While it's common for some Finnish people to enjoy a gin drink, known as a "Long Drink" or "Lonkero," during a sauna session, it is best to steer clear of alcohol immediately before, during, and after your sauna session.
- Individuals taking medications that impact their thermoregulation, such as antipsychotics, antihistamines, antidepressants, and beta-blockers, should exercise caution when using a sauna as they may be at an increased risk of heat stroke.
- Sauna use is not recommended for children, pregnant women, elderly individuals with low blood pressure, or those who have recently had a heart attack.

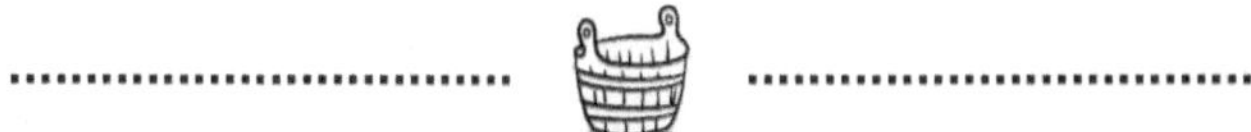

CHAPTER FOUR

TYPES

Purists claim that the traditional dry sauna is the only "true" sauna, but the comparative benefits of different sauna types remain inconclusive. Most studies focus on either traditional or infrared saunas individually, making it difficult to determine which offers more benefits. However, heat stress from any form of sauna, or even hot bath, can provide benefits and activate heat shock proteins (HSPs) (more on HSPs and their benefits in the next chapter). The specific benefits may vary depending on the type.

Traditional Dry Sauna

- Traditional dry saunas have been studied more

extensively, so some experts consider them the "safer" choice.

- People who are more sensitive to heat may find the temperature overwhelming.

Infrared Sauna

- There is more limited research to support infrared saunas. Most sauna studies used a temperature of at least 174°F, but infrared saunas cannot reach that level. Point blank, many experts say infrared saunas don't get hot enough.
- Infrared saunas can be more comfortable because they don't get as hot as traditional saunas. This lower temperature allows you to stay inside longer without feeling too hot.
- The infrared sauna industry can sometimes be heavily influenced by marketing.
- Some people have raised concerns about the potential electromagnetic field (EMF) risks with certain types of infrared saunas, but no medical evidence of harmful effects exists. Some infrared sauna companies offer EMF testing or use methods to minimize EMFs.

Steam Room

- Similar to infrared saunas, steam rooms do not get hot enough.
- The high humidity does not allow sweat to evaporate off the skin, thus making it a bit harder on your heart.

If you do not have access to a sauna, another great option for heat stress is actually submerging in a very hot bath or jacuzzi (around 104°F) up to your shoulders. In one small study, participants who stayed in a hot bath for about 30 minutes saw improvements in depressive symptoms and sleep quality (Naumann et al., 2017). In another hot bath study, HSP levels increased by around 40% (compared to 50% during a sauna) (Faulkner et al., 2017).

PART 2
BENEFITS

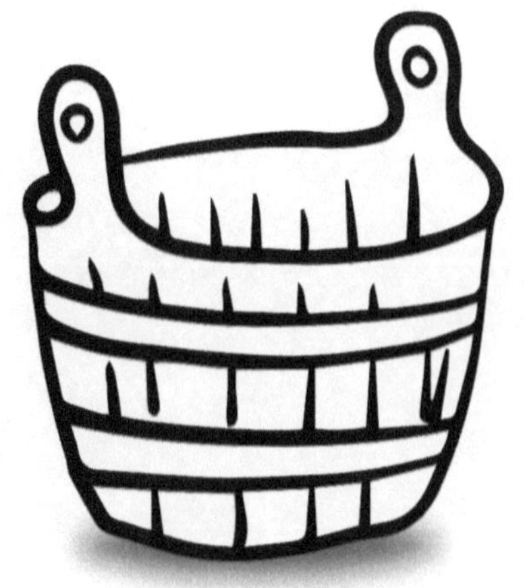

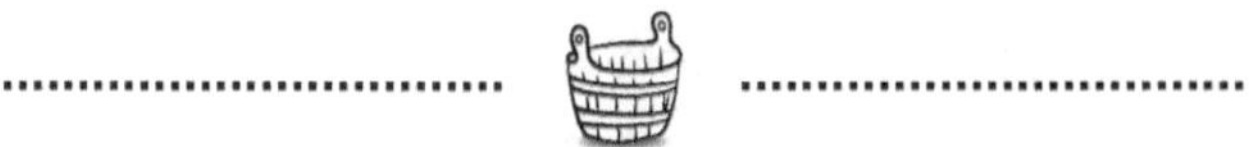

HEAT SHOCK PROTEINS

This is the most scientific we'll get, so bear with me! You'll see the term HSPs come up a lot. In short, HSPs make healthy cells stronger and protect against diseases. They are activated in response to heat stress. Now, let's clarify, a little bit of stress is actually beneficial for the body.

Humans are built to activate our stress pathways. Historically, we naturally experienced stress through activities like foraging and hunting. In our modern world, where instant gratification is the norm, we often lack these natural stressors.

That's where strategies like exercise, intermittent fasting, and even heat exposure, such as sauna bathing, come into play. By engaging in these practices, we can stimulate the production of HSPs and enjoy their potential benefits, including preventing muscle atrophy, mitigating neurodegenerative diseases, and reducing arterial plaques. And on top of this, heat can elicit a powerful antioxidant and anti-inflammatory response.

- HSPs can prevent muscle loss and protect against neurodegenerative diseases (Leak, 2014).
- Heat stress, like saunas, is especially effective at increasing HSP levels. Within 30 minutes, HSP levels can increase by up to 49% (Yamada et al., 2007; Iguchi et al., 2012).
- These increased HSP levels are sustained over time, especially in heat-adapted individuals.

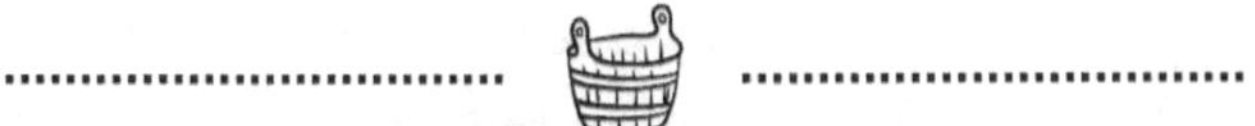

CHAPTER SIX

CARDIOVASCULAR HEALTH

Regular sauna sessions, specifically more than 4 times a week, have been found to significantly reduce the risk of sudden cardiac death and fatal cardiovascular events. The heat from the sauna increases body temperature, thus improving blood flow, cardiac output, and the dilation of blood vessels. These combined effects make sauna sessions a potential game-changer for heart health.

- During a sauna, cardiac output can increase as much as 70% (Hannuksela & Ellahham, 2001).
- Heart rate can rise to 150 beats per minute, mimicking moderate-intensity exercise (Ketelhut, 2019).

- Multiple studies have indicated that regular sauna bathing (four to seven times per week) can lower the risk of fatal heart disease by approximately 50%, sudden cardiac death by 60%, stroke by 51%, and hypertension by 46%.
- Frequent sauna sessions can lower the risk of cardiovascular disease by up to 63% (Laukkanen et al., 2015).
- Participants who used saunas two to three times per week had a 24% lower risk of all-cause mortality, while those who used saunas four to seven times per week had a 40% lower chance (Laukkanen et al., 2015).

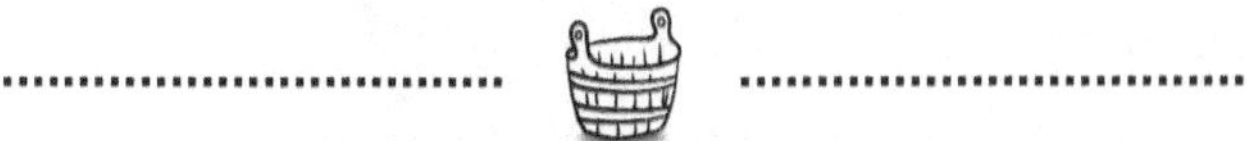

CHAPTER SEVEN

RESPIRATORY HEALTH

"The sauna is a poor man's pharmacy" is a Finnish proverb highlighting saunas' remarkable health benefits. They have been found to reduce the risk of pulmonary diseases like pneumonia, asthma, and chronic obstructive pulmonary disease (COPD) by modulating the immune system. Sauna sessions increase the counts of important immune cells, such as white blood cells, lymphocytes, and neutrophils (Pilch et al., 2013). HSPs also play a crucial role in preserving immunological resilience.

As a reminder, traditional saunas and steam rooms have higher humidity levels, whereas infrared saunas have no humidity and may not offer the same respiratory benefits.

- Saunas can have a protective effect against the common cold. However, it took three months of usage before the sauna had a protective effect (Ernst et al., 1990).
- Participants who engaged in sauna sessions two to three times per week had a 27% lower likelihood of developing pneumonia than those who rarely or never used saunas. Additionally, individuals who participated in over four weekly sauna sessions experienced a 41% reduced risk of pneumonia (Kunutsor et al., 2017).

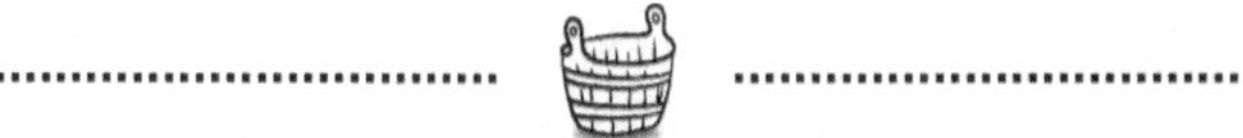

CHAPTER EIGHT

COGNITIVE FUNCTION

According to Dr. Jari Laukakken, frequent sauna sessions are linked to a lower risk of dementia and Alzheimer's disease. As discussed previously, a sauna triggers the activation of HSPs, which play a vital role in cellular repair and maintenance. By protecting against the accumulation of misfolded proteins and the formation of amyloid plaques, HSPs help safeguard against Alzheimer's.

- Those who used the sauna once per week had a 21% lower risk for dementia, whereas those who used it four to seven times per week had a 66% lower chance (Laukkanen et al., 2016).
- Alzheimer's risk was 20% lower for individuals

who used the sauna once per week and 65% lower for those who used it four to seven times per week (Laukkanen et al., 2016).

- Sauna use was associated with improved cognitive function, including memory, attention, and processing speed (Cernych et al., 2018).

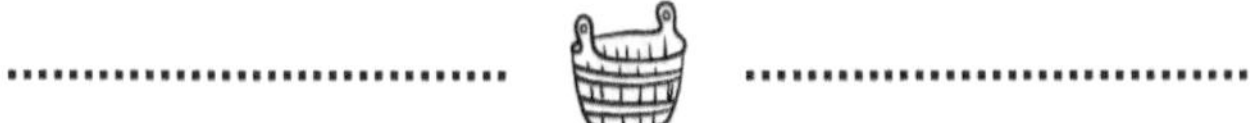

CHAPTER NINE

MENTAL HEALTH

Saunas work wonders for our mood and stress levels. They help reduce cortisol, the stress hormone, and trigger the release of euphoric hormones like serotonin, norepinephrine, dopamine, and oxytocin. This creates an antidepressant effect, temporarily relieving stress and boosting our overall mood.

- Sauna use decreased depression symptoms, improved appetite, and reduced anxiety and body aches (Masuda et al., 2005).
- Just one sauna session showed depressive symptoms decrease by 50%, with the benefits persisting for six weeks (Janssen et al., 2016).
- Sauna bathing can lower cortisol, your body's

stress hormone, by 10–40% (Leppaluoto et al., 1986; Kukkonen-Harjula et al.,1989).

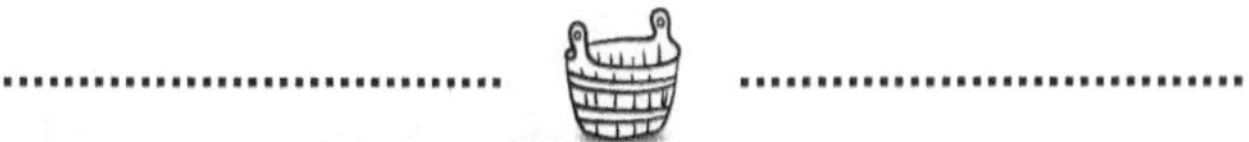

CHAPTER TEN

GROWTH HORMONE

Sauna use has a fascinating effect on growth hormone levels in the body, which can lead to a range of benefits, including improved muscle mass, bone density, and sleep.

The release of growth hormone is temperature and duration dependent and not suitable for everyone. To maximize growth hormone effects, Dr. Andrew Huberman says to sauna once a week or less, with four 30-minute sessions and cooldown periods in between. Enter the sauna in a fasted state, avoiding food for two to three hours prior.

It's worth mentioning that the increase in growth hormone levels induced by saunas is typically temporary, returning to normal after a few hours.

- Two sauna sessions at 176°F (80°C), each lasting 20 minutes and separated by a 30-minute cooling period, resulted in a 100% increase in growth hormone levels compared to baseline. In contrast, two sauna sessions at 212°F (100°C), each lasting 15 minutes and separated by a 30-minute cooling period, led to a 500% increase in growth hormone levels (Hannuksela & Ellahham, 2001; Kukkonen-Harjula et al., 1989).

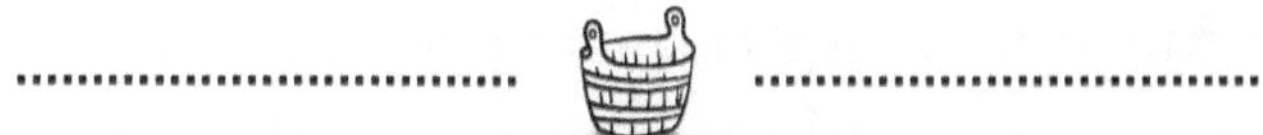

CHAPTER ELEVEN

SLEEP

Getting quality sleep is essential for overall health and functioning. Poor sleep can impair brain function and contribute to a range of health problems, from cognitive decline to weakened immunity and mental health disorders.

Both body temperature and hormones play a vital role in regulating sleep. Falling asleep requires your core body temperature to cool down by around 1-3°F. After an evening sauna session, your body naturally starts to cool off, signaling that it's time to wind down for sleep. As we now know, saunas also stimulate the release of growth hormone, which has a direct impact on sleep.

For the best results, sauna in the early evening to

allow your body enough time to cool down before bed.

- Growth hormone can increase slow-wave sleep, or deep sleep, which is the most restorative sleep stage (Wilckens et al., 2018).
- Saunas can increase deep sleep by up to 70%. During the first few hours, deep sleep increased by 70%, and after six hours, there was still a 45% increase (Putkonen & Elomaa, 1976).
- Heat therapy can help with increased deep sleep, 'good sleep', and 'quickness of falling asleep' (Bunnell et al., 1988; Liao, 2022).

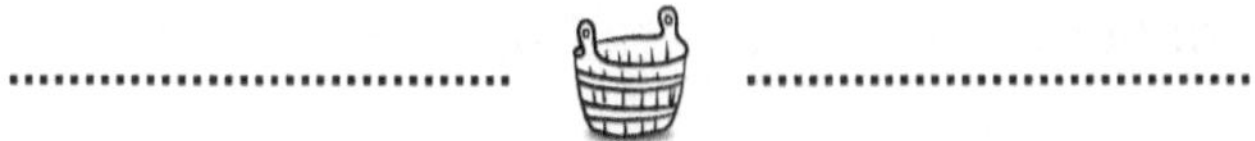

INSULIN SENSITIVITY

Have you heard of insulin sensitivity? It refers to how effectively our bodies can use sugar for energy. Even if you're not dealing with diabetes, understanding this can shed light on your overall health.

Let's break it down: Our bodies naturally produce a hormone called insulin. When we eat, especially foods rich in carbohydrates, our digestive system breaks down what we've eaten into glucose (sugar). This glucose enters our bloodstream, causing our pancreas (a gland behind the stomach) to release insulin into the blood. If our bodies are insulin-sensitive, we can maintain stable blood sugar levels and reduce our risk of diabetes and metabolic disorders. If we are insulin resistant, excess glucose accumulates in the body, contributing to weight gain and fat storage. It can also disrupt the hormones in metabolism, potentially leading to increased hunger and overeating.

All that science mumbo jumbo to say that sauna use increases insulin sensitivity and helps manage glucose control, largely through the increased levels of HSPs.

- When insulin-resistant mice were exposed to heat therapy three times a week for 12 weeks, their blood glucose levels decreased, and their plasma insulin levels dropped by 31%, suggesting improved insulin sensitivity (Kokura et al., 2007).

CHAPTER THIRTEEN

ATHLETIC PERFORMANCE

When you sauna regularly, exercise can actually become easier. Why is that? Well, becoming heat adaptive increases your plasma volume, blood flow, and oxygen availability to your muscles. That means less relative stress on your lungs or heart. On top of that, if you can cool off easier (or sweat at a lower body temperature), then you will delay fatigue and be able to work harder for longer. As we already know, saunas are also great for increasing levels of HSPs and growth hormones, which directly impact muscle growth, repair, and maintenance.

For optimal results, use the sauna after your workout instead of before to maximize its benefits.

- Participants who used a sauna after exercise showed improved endurance and faster recovery times. One study found that a 30-minute sauna session following training increased endurance capacity by 32% compared to exercise alone (Laukkanen et al., 2015).
- Sauna use can help prevent muscle loss (Ihsan et al., 2020).

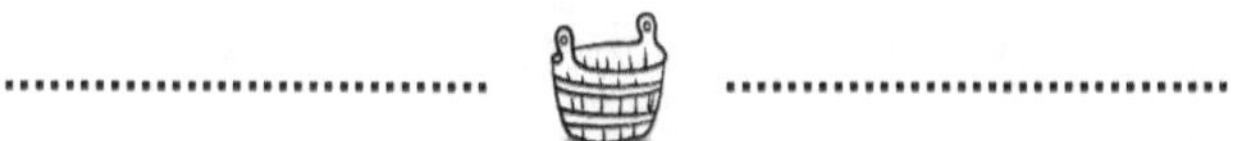

DETOXIFICATION

Many people believe that saunas help the body detoxify, but it's important to understand why. Saunas make you sweat, and sweating is a natural way for the body to get rid of waste and toxins. However, the idea that saunas are a powerful detox method is often exaggerated. In reality, the liver and kidneys are the body's main organs for detoxification. Interestingly, despite this, certain heavy metals, such as lead and cadmium, are excreted in higher concentrations through sweat compared to urine.

Why does this matter? Well, some level of heavy metal contamination in your life is inevitable. While certain metals like iron are essential for good health, others, such as lead and cadmium, can be harmful when present in significant amounts. These heavy metals can enter the body through food and polluted water, air, and everyday items. They may naturally occur in soil and enter the food chain or be introduced through human activities like farming. For instance, lead can leach into drinking water from lead pipes and may be found in imported pottery. Cadmium can naturally occur in the environment or be introduced through industrial activities and can contaminate crops, especially shellfish, grains, and leafy greens. Heavy metal exposure can have serious consequences. High cadmium levels are linked to increased breast cancer risk, while elevated lead levels are a serious concern for pregnant women and children.

- Dr. Rhonda Patrick says the average person loses about 1.1 pounds of sweat during a sauna session. This is due to the increased cardiac output and blood flow distribution to the skin.
- Lead is eliminated through sweat at a rate 14 times higher than that observed in urine, while cadmium is excreted in sweat at a rate 11 times greater than in urine.

PART 3
DISADVANTAGES

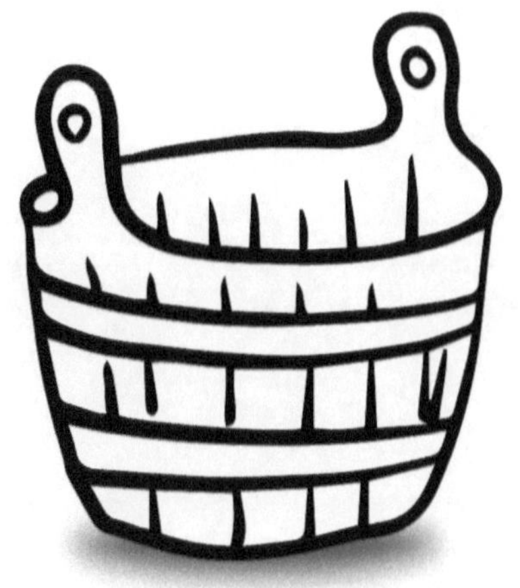

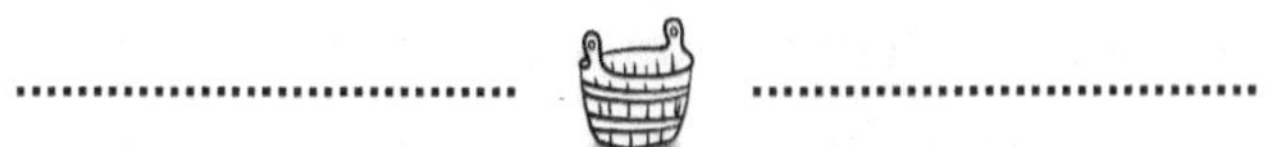

CHAPTER FIFTEEN

FERTILITY

While you should not expect immediate elimination of all sperm from a sauna visit, the heat generated by saunas can potentially harm sperm and impede sperm production, particularly with regular sauna use. The optimal conditions for healthy sperm production involve maintaining a scrotal temperature 2-3°F degrees lower than the body temperature. Elevating the temperature of the scrotum and testes by a few degrees can harm sperm production and sperm health. Of course, it's important to note that even the heat from hot tubs can damage sperm too.

- Lower sperm counts and decreased sperm

motility were observed in individuals who used the sauna for 15 minutes twice a week over three months. However, these results seem to be temporary. Three months after discontinuing sauna visits, the sperm counts remained below average, but after six months, the sperm counts returned to normal levels (Garolla et al., 2013).

- Even one 20-minute session at 185°F (86°C) was shown to alter sperm mitochondria, which are responsible for cellular energy production and sperm motility. Within one week of the exposure, there was a decline in sperm count, which subsequently returned to normal levels within five weeks (Huhtaniemi & Laukkanen, 2020).

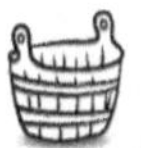

FAQS

Now, let's be honest — this book may not address every pressing question you have about saunas. The research on saunas is still relatively new, so not all benefits have been conclusively proven through scientific studies. For those remaining questions, I've gathered the most impartial and reputable answers available.

Should I eat before a sauna?
- It's best to have a light snack, like fruit, before a sauna. You should not sauna with a full or empty stomach as it could lead to discomfort, dizziness, or nausea.

Should I drink water during a sauna?

- While some discourage consuming water during the sauna to maintain the body's detoxification process, scientific evidence does not validate this notion. Generally, you should be well-hydrated before a sauna session and can sip warm water as needed during the session to replenish lost fluids. After the sauna, aim to consume two to four glasses of water for optimal rehydration.

Can saunas benefit my skin?

- Regular sauna sessions can cleanse pores and improve circulation for a healthier complexion. However, caution is advised for individuals with psoriasis or eczema, as sauna heat can exacerbate symptoms. If you have sensitive skin, opting for a steam room may be a better choice than a dry or infrared sauna, as the humid environment is generally gentler. Make sure to hydrate and moisturize after a sauna session to help alleviate any dryness. Always consult a dermatologist for personalized advice.

Can saunas damage hair?

- Saunas can potentially have adverse effects on your hair. The high heat and low moisture levels can lead to dryness and make hair more brittle. However, this concern mainly applies to extended sauna sessions or existing hair issues. To protect your hair, consider using a hair mask or deep conditioning treatment before entering the sauna, staying hydrated, covering your hair with a cap or towel, and rinse with cool water post-sauna.

Can I lose weight from saunas?

- Saunas can lead to temporary weight loss through sweating, but it's important to understand that this weight loss is primarily water weight and not fat loss. Relying solely on saunas is not an effective long-term weight loss approach. While the increase in heart rate and sweating in a sauna can burn some calories, it's not a substitute for regular exercise in terms of calorie expenditure. Nevertheless, saunas can play a supportive role in weight management by boosting insulin sensitivity and helping regulate glucose levels.

Do saunas help hangovers?

- Saunas may offer some relief for hangovers by increasing circulation and aiding in detoxification through sweating. However, they are only a partial solution. Hangovers often come with dehydration, which can be exacerbated by saunas. Combine sauna use with other hangover remedies for the best results, prioritizing rehydration and rest.

Why do some sauna enthusiasts wear hats in the sauna?

- Your head tends to overheat first, so a sauna hat acts as a barrier from the heat. It prevents your scalp, hair, and ears from becoming uncomfortable, ensuring longer sauna sessions. Additionally, it can protect color-treated hair, from potential heat-induced damage and can reduce the chance of split ends. Traditionally, these hats are crafted from materials like wool felt.

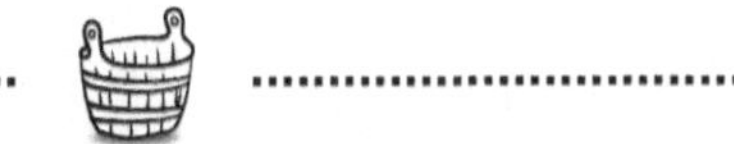

FURTHER READING

If you enjoyed *Saunas Simplified*, stay tuned for the next book release on the power of cold therapy to reduce stress, inflammation, and more.

REFERENCES

Beever R (2009). Far-infrared saunas for treatment of cardiovascular risk factors: summary of published evidence. Can Fam Physician 55, 7.

Bunnell, D. E., Agnew, J. A., Horvath, S. M., Jopson, L., & Wills, M. (1988). Passive body heating and sleep: Influence of proximity to sleep. Sleep, 11(2), 210–219.

Cernych, M., Satas, A., & Brazaitis, M. (2018). Post-sauna recovery enhances brain neural network relaxation and improves cognitive economy in oddball tasks. International Journal of Hyperthermia 35(1), 375–382.

Ernst, E., Pecho, E., Wirz, P., & Saradeth, T. (1990). Regular sauna bathing and the incidence of common colds. Annals of Medicine, 22(4), 225–227.

Faulkner, S. H., Jackson, S., Fatania, G., & Leicht, C. A. (2017). The effect of passive heating on heat shock protein 70 and interleukin-6: A possible treatment tool for metabolic diseases? Temperature, 4(3), 292–304.

Garolla, A., Torino, M., Sartini, B., Cosci, I., Patassini, C., Carraro, U., & Foresta, C. (2013). Seminal and molecular evidence that sauna exposure affects human spermatogenesis. Human Reproduction, 28(4), 877–885.

Hannuksela, M. L., & Ellahham, S. (2001). Benefits and risks of Sauna Bathing. The American Journal of Medicine, 110(2), 118–126.

Huhtaniemi, I. T., & Laukkanen, J. A. (2020). Endocrine effects of Sauna Bath. Current Opinion in Endocrine and Metabolic Research, 11, 15–20.

Ihsan, M., Deldicque, L., Molphy, J., Britto, F., Cherif, A., & Racinais, S. (2020). Skeletal muscle signaling following whole-body and localized heat exposure in humans. Frontiers in Physiology, 11.

Janssen, C. W., Lowry, C. A., Mehl, M. R., Allen, J. J.,
Kelly, K. L., Gartner, D. E., Medrano, A., Begay, T.
K., Rentscher, K., White, J. J., Fridman, A., Roberts,
L. J., Robbins, M. L., Hanusch, K., Cole, S. P., &
Raison, C. L. (2016). Whole-body hyperthermia for
the treatment of major depressive disorder. JAMA
Psychiatry, 73(8), 789.

Ketelhut, S., & Ketelhut, R. G. (2019). The blood
pressure and heart rate during sauna bath
correspond to cardiac responses during submaximal
dynamic exercise. Complementary Therapies in
Medicine, 44, 218–222.

Kokura, S., Adachi, S., Manabe, E., Mizushima, K.,
Hattori, T., Okuda, T., Nakabe, N., Handa, O.,
Takagi, T., Naito, Y., Yoshida, N., & Yoshikawa, T.
(2007). Whole body hyperthermia improves obesity-
induced insulin resistance in diabetic mice.
International Journal of Hyperthermia, 23(3), 259–
265.

Kukkonen-Harjula, K., & Kauppinen, K. (2006). Health
effects and risks of Sauna Bathing. International
Journal of Circumpolar Health, 65(3), 195–205.

Kukkonen-Harjula, K., Oja, P., Laustiola, K., Vuori, I.,
Jolkkonen, J., Siitonen, S., & Vapaatalo, H. (1989).

Haemodynamic and hormonal responses to heat exposure in a finnish sauna bath. European Journal of Applied Physiology and Occupational Physiology, 58(5), 543–550.

Kunutsor, S. K., Laukkanen, T., & Laukkanen, J. A. (2017). Sauna bathing reduces the risk of respiratory diseases: A long-term prospective cohort study. European Journal of Epidemiology, 32(12), 1107–1111.

Laukkanen, T., Khan, H., Zaccardi, F., & Laukkanen, J. A. (2015). Association between sauna bathing and fatal cardiovascular and all-cause mortality events. JAMA Internal Medicine, 175(4), 542.

Laukkanen, T., Kunutsor, S., Kauhanen, J., & Laukkanen, J. A. (2016). Sauna bathing is inversely associated with dementia and alzheimer's disease 65(3), 195–205.

Leak, R. K. (2014). Heat shock proteins in neurodegenerative disorders and aging. Journal of Cell Communication and Signaling, 8(4), 293–310.

Leppäluoto, J., Huttunen, P., Hirvonen, J., Väänänen, A., Tuominen, M., & Vuori, J. (1986). Endocrine effects of repeated sauna bathing. Acta Physiologica

Scandinavica, 128(3), 467–470.

Liao, W.-C. (2002). Effects of passive body heating on body temperature and sleep regulation in the elderly: A systematic review. International Journal of Nursing Studies, 39(8), 803–810.

Masuda, A., Nakazato, M., Kihara, T., Minagoe, S., & Tei, C. (2005). Repeated thermal therapy diminishes appetite loss and subjective complaints in mildly depressed patients. Psychosomatic Medicine, 67(4), 643–647.

Naumann, J., Grebe, J., Kaifel, S., Weinert, T., Sadaghiani, C., & Huber, R. (2017). Effects of hyperthermic baths on depression, sleep and heart rate variability in patients with depressive disorder: A randomized clinical pilot trial. BMC Complementary and Alternative Medicine, 17(1).

Pilch, W., Szyguła, Z., Palka, T., Pilch, P., Cison, T., Wiecha, S., & Tota, Ł. (2014). Comparison of physiological reactions and physiological strain in healthy men under heat stress in dry and steam heat saunas. Biology of Sport, 31(2), 145–149.

Putkonen, P.T.S., Eloma, E., (1976). Sauna and physiological sleep: Increased slow-wave sleep after heat exposure. Sauna Studies. pp 270-279. Vammala. ISBN: 951-95328-0-3

Wilckens, K. A., Ferrarelli, F., Walker, M. P., & Buysse, D. J. (2018). Slow-wave activity enhancement to improve cognition. Trends in Neurosciences, 41(7), 470–482.

Yamada, P. M., Amorim, F. T., Moseley, P., Robergs, R., & Schneider, S. M. (2007). Effect of heat acclimation on heat shock protein 72 and interleukin-10 in humans. Journal of Applied Physiology, 103(4), 1196–1204.